Fractured Silence

Also by Margaret A. Jones and published by Ginninderra Press
The Lost Child

Margaret A. Jones
& Rachel Ferneley

Fractured Silence

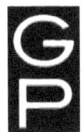

Fractured Silence
ISBN 978 1 74027 840 9
Copyright © text Margaret A. Jones @ Rachel Ferneley 2013
Cover painting: Rachel Ferneley

First published 2013
Reprinted 2016

GINNINDERRA PRESS
PO Box 3461 Port Adelaide 5015
www.ginninderrapress.com.au

Contents

Introduction		7
Part One Margaret's Story		9
1	First things	11
2	Epiphany	16
3	The arrival	19
4	The diagnosis	24
5	Practicalities	28
6	Other side effects	30
7	Early training	34
8	Battle of wills	39
9	Early schooling	42
10	Our new life in Australia	45
11	Penshurst Opportunity for the Deaf Unit	47
12	New beginnings	51
13	Danny	54
Part Two Rachel's Story		57
Being deaf		59
Postscript		75
Appendix		76

Introduction

This is the story of my struggle to bring language to my child, who was born with a severe hearing loss as a result of congenital rubella. It is also the same story as experienced by my daughter and told in her own words. Our stories show readers how courage and determination can overcome such a difficult disability

We have written our story firstly to help the general public understand what it means to be born deaf and hopefully build a better understanding between both the hearing and deaf cultures. We also hope our story may help other families who have, or are now having, similar problems; from our experiences they will take heart and know that, however difficult it all seems, there is a light at the end of the tunnel.

Margaret

Part One

Margaret's Story

1

First things

On an auspicious day in March 1962, I slipped out of work to keep an appointment with the gynaecologist who was going to tell me whether I was pregnant or not.

After the examination, the young doctor looked steadily at me for a moment while peeling off his gloves. 'You are,' he said at last. 'Is this good news, or bad?'

I had just turned twenty but looked more like a child of fifteen; hence his question, I suppose. My squeal of joy gave him his answer.

'Oh, I see! Well then, go home and tell your husband your good news.'

I left the hospital in a dream. All I had ever wanted was to have my own child. When I was just a slip of a girl, I pestered the mothers in my street to take their babies for a walk, and there were plenty to choose from in the Glasgow tenements. Invariably the mothers happily agreed. I expect they were only too grateful to have a break from one of their many offspring. For me, though, it was magical.

When I held a little child close to me, my own life faded and all that was real and good emanated from these little creatures and from the bright eyes smiling at me, and the wee, fat hands patting my cheek, or pulling at my nose. To them I was just another human they had to touch and explore and smile at because I was smiling at them and making silly noises, but to me they were as beautiful and spectacular to behold as diamonds are to other girls. Now, I was going to have my very own!

The ground hardly stayed beneath my feet as I made my way back to work. Instead of taking the bus, I walked the couple of miles to stretch out the moments in which to savour my own special joy; to keep the knowledge safely locked within myself for as long as possible before the spell must break and I would have to share it with my husband, David, and waiting colleagues.

My older sister, Pat, who lived nearby, would of course have to be told, though that would be later. Pat was expecting her fourth child in five years; understandably my news wouldn't be met with quite the same excitement and pleasure as I would, selfishly, have liked it to be – you know, big hugs, cheers and celebrations – so I held off telling her.

I was seven weeks pregnant before I decided to share my news with Pat. It was on a cold and wet Tuesday evening.

After dinner I said to David, 'Let's go and visit Pat and Mike.'

He gave a small smile. 'And tell them your good news, I presume!'

'You presume right,' I said, smiling widely.

It was around eight o'clock when we arrived on their doorstep.

My sister opened the door and greeted us with her lovely, bright smile. 'Margaret! David! Hello. Come on in out of the cold and wet.'

We went in. All three children were in bed upstairs so we had the living room to ourselves. Pat made us tea.

It was while sitting around the fire chatting together that she suddenly announced, 'Young Mike's got German measles. If I get it, I'll have to have this one aborted.'

'Why's that, Pat?' I gasped in horror.

'Because it could be damaged.'

Her reply sent me reeling. 'How? In what way?'

'It could be blind or deaf, or both. Or worse. I'm only just twelve weeks. After three months it's not so serious because all their nerves and vital organs have developed by then.'

Her reply seemed so clinical and matter-of-fact. I felt my insides churning, I wanted to scream. But all I could manage to say was 'I hope you don't get it.'

It seemed pointless now to share my joyful news with my sister.

There was now no joy; that feeling had been replaced with a skimpy little hope that, since young Michael was upstairs, I wouldn't catch the virus.

Three weeks later, I woke up with a fever and face and neck full of bright red spots. I went to my doctor.

He looked at the spots and felt behind my ears for the telltale lumps. He nodded. 'You have rubella.'

I looked puzzled; I hadn't heard that word before.

'German measles,' he added casually before turning towards his prescription pad.

My reaction made him stop and swivel back to me. There was concern in his eyes, I could tell, for I was screaming, 'My baby is being damaged, my baby is being damaged.'

He rose and walked to his medicine cupboard. 'I'll give you an injection of gamma globulin. It will help fight the virus,' he said. He injected me with the medication and told me to go home and rest while reassuring me that my baby would be all right and that I should try not to worry.

I could not go home and rest. Instead I took a taxi to my sister Pat's home and told her then about my pregnancy and the rubella. We were standing by her fireplace. I was looking at her reflection in the mirror; I had never seen her look so shocked.

'Oh, Margaret! Why didn't you tell me you were pregnant?' She sat me down beside her on the sofa. Her hazel eyes stared solemnly into mine. 'I think you should have it aborted,' she advised softly.

We both knew abortions were illegal. Women resorted to backyard abortions or self-induced miscarriages all the time. In our street it was a common thing. A vision leapt into my mind of a young neighbour who I walked in on one day when I was about sixteen. Apparently she had tried to self-abort and it had failed. I found her lying prostrate on the bed crying out for her mother. On the floor there stood a bucket half-filled with her blood with the foetus still clinging stubbornly to life inside her. Then there was the frantic dash to hospital to have her womb scraped and life saved.

'I'll have to think about it, Pat. Remember Janice next door?'

'Yes. I know. That poor girl. The miscarriage mucked up her insides. She couldn't get pregnant when she wanted one later on.' My sister looked thoughtfully into the distance then smiled ironically. 'I have no trouble getting pregnant.'

She leaned her elbows on her knees and cupped her chin in her hands. Dark circles under her eyes had become a part of my sister as had her constant tiredness. 'Anyway,' she said firmly, 'there's a new pill coming out that stops women getting pregnant. I'll be taking it after this one – for the rest of my fertile life.'

We fell silent, both lost in our own thoughts. Things had changed between us now. I had always looked upon Pat as my second mother. She was the eldest of my mother's brood of seven and, at a young age, had been forced to shoulder the responsibility of caring for us when our mother became clinically depressed. Now, though, I was no longer a child. I was a woman faced with a woman's problem – just like millions of other women, including my own mother and sisters. This was a decision I would have to make by myself.

'What did the doctor say? Did he offer to give you an abortion?' she asked at last.

'No. He gave me an injection to help fight off the virus. Gamma globulin he called it. Told me to go home and rest and not to worry as my baby would be all right.'

'What!' Pat's intake of breath told me what she thought about that.

'What's the matter with that?' I asked, alarmed.

'I can't see how it would have helped, that's all.'

'Like closing the stable door after the horse has bolted, you mean.'

'Something like that.' She sighed deeply.

'It wouldn't harm it, though – would it?'

She shrugged. 'Shouldn't think so. It's just a bit late for it, that's all, unfortunately.'

'So, what is gamma globulin, Pat?'

'Well, *Gamma Glo*bulin injections are usually given to try to temporarily boost the immune system against disease. The doctor probably just gave you it to make you feel a bit less distressed. That's all.'

After a while she asked, 'What are you going to do now?'

'I don't know. I'll have to think about it for a bit.'

She heaved a sigh. 'I don't envy you. It won't be an easy decision. God knows I know just how hard it will be.'

As I was leaving, she gave me an unaccustomed quick hug. 'Don't take too long,' she advised. 'The sooner it's done, the better it will be for you.'

2

Epiphany

I don't remember how I got home but I will not forget the next few days. David, as silent and uncommunicative as always, was even less able to support me. I stayed alone in the dark and dingy room we had rented, alone with my thoughts and feelings. Being a very emotional girl, I felt overcome with grief and cried for what seemed like an eternity.

When at last it stopped, I went to the mirror and looked at myself. A young face, still showing puppy fat, stared wide-eyed back at me. For the first time, I understood pain in all its grotesque proportions.

When I was a child, there was a deaf boy in my class. He was silent and seemingly unfriendly. One day a group of my school friends and I talked about what would be worse – being deaf or blind; if we had to be one or the other, which one would we choose? I never could decide, for they were both equally as horrible to imagine. Now I was faced with the question again.

If my child was going to be deaf, how would this affect its life? I thought of the hours of pleasure I had experienced when listening to beautiful music. My child would never know that pleasure. Birdsong would mean nothing, nor would it hear the wind in the trees, or water bubbling in a stream or crashing on the shore; never hear my words, or know what a crowd of people were laughing and chattering about, never know what was being said on the television, or in a schoolroom. What kind of person would it become without knowing these things, and being denied spiritual nourishment from these compensatory gifts of nature?

Or what if it was going to be blind? I closed my eyes and thought of what it would miss out on. It would never be thrilled by the beauty of a sunset, or gasp at the splendour of a great tree swaying in the wind, or the sun sparkling on an expanse of water, or appreciate the exquisite beauty of the colours and shapes of flowers. All of nature's immense creations would be as nothing to my child. What would it be like not to know my face, or recognise another human being, see a smile, or be aware of a dangerous obstacle in its path? Or know the pleasure and freedom of being able to drive oneself about?

I could not continue to contemplate how this would affect my child, or whether I could cope with the sadness that would follow my every waking hour when I thought of the treasures this virus had stolen from it.

My thoughts turned to myself and my husband. We were at the start of our life together, a life that could produce abundant healthy children. Would it be wrong to choose to start again, with a healthy child? Or was it selfish and cruel not to give this child a chance now that it had been started? I was twenty years old and faced with this terrible, moral dilemma.

For the next two days I sat alone, thinking about my future and the choice I would have to make. I wonder now as I write why I did not share these thoughts with anyone – not even my own mother? Or why my husband did not discuss it with me. I seem to remember being totally alone with the problem and having to make the decision all by myself.

*

I finally made up my mind to have the child aborted. Not as a backyard job, but in a hospital where I would be safe. I knew abortions were illegal but surely, for reasons such as a definite physical threat to a child, an exception would be made in my case. My intelligence and common sense told me that I ought to be successful. In any case, I would insist. I would not leave the hospital until they agreed to do it.

*

It was while walking past the local church, crying to myself, that I became aware of a voice calling out to me from within the church grounds. I turned and saw that it belonged to an old lady. She called me over to the gate and asked me why I was crying. I told her where I was going and what I intended to do.

She looked intently at me for a moment then in a cool, clear tone said, 'My dear, you could be destroying the most beautiful person. Do you really want to do that?'

Her words cut through my misery and embedded themselves in my soul. I gazed at her and held onto her now shining eyes while my universe realigned. I looked over her shoulder at the church. It was glowing with soft, spring sunlight, imbuing it with a feeling of gentleness and enduring strength. Something shifted inside me. I suddenly realised the tight band around my chest had loosened and I felt able to breath properly.

It is difficult to explain my feelings from this distance in time, except to say the dread at what might happen disintegrated and a new feeling of confidence and optimism grew steadily in my heart. I felt instinctively I was receiving a message from God. When I returned my eyes to the woman, I no longer saw just an old woman dressed in black, but a spiritual presence – God's emissary, if you like. For a long moment we stood together in silence, each conscious that the life of another being rested precariously on the edge of a moral and ethical choice.

At last I took a deep breath, looked steadily into her eyes and uttered the words that would change my life forever. 'I won't go to the hospital.'

She said quietly, 'God bless you and take care of you both.'

I turned around and walked back to the flat. On the way I placed my hand on my stomach and said to my child, 'You're going to be all right. God is going to help us.

3

The arrival

Once the decision was made to keep the baby, I got back to my normal life and tried to put negative thoughts out of my head. I wanted to reclaim my former joy at having my very own child. The experience at the church had filled me with a sure knowledge that whatever might be affected by the virus this child was blessed by God and would consequently have a good life.

*

One day, four months into the pregnancy, while sitting on the sofa and leaning forward to get a cup from the coffee table, I felt a fluttering against my groin. My baby had kicked me! It was alive and growing! My joy returned tenfold. It was a long time between kicks as this child seemed to want to sleep all the time. However, there was enough movement to keep me happy.

In September, Pat gave birth to her fourth child and third daughter; a blonde, blue-eyed cutie they named Hilary. When I held her in my arms and kissed her soft, pink cheek, my heart leapt with excitement; I couldn't wait for my very own child to arrive.

My baby was due in early November. On the nominated date, I had contractions and went to hospital. Nothing happened and they sent me home again telling me to wait until the waters broke. For almost three long weeks, the child refused to arrive. In the end, nineteen days after the due date, they took me in to be induced the next morning. During the night, my daughter decided to upstage them and began her journey into this world at three a.m. I was taken to the labour ward, but again it all stopped. At eight a.m. they decided to induce me after all. Before doing so, they very kindly supplied me with a dose of pethidine and I was wheeled into the delivery room in a high state of intoxication. At one-twenty p.m. on 20 November 1962, Rachel Harriet was born.

The birth itself was relatively painless. The child slipped out in one great, satisfying push. But I heard no crying and saw they had taken her to a side table and were working on her body, rubbing it until she coughed and whimpered. They assured me she was all right, just a little sleepy. Without even showing me my child, or letting me hold her, they wrapped her up and took her away. I was told they would bring her to me after I had had a rest.

My imagination, of course, was running riot. Was there something wrong with her? Had she been rushed to the operating theatre? Why wasn't I being told anything at all? They knew I was worried because she was a rubella baby. Didn't they understand this and offer me some reassurance? My lifelong feelings of anxiety were born along with Rachel, simply because no one was telling me anything.

They brought my baby to me in the late afternoon. She was fast asleep and very pale. A little hot water bottle lay alongside her – because, they said, she was cold. I got to hold this precious bundle for the very first time. I examined her all over, as all mothers do. Her skin was wrinkled and peeling because of being well overdue. She had a great birthmark on her forehead and over her eye. This alarmed me until I was told it was a strawberry stain caused by the pressure of being locked in the birth canal for some time. (Now I know it is a rubella symptom called 'blueberry bun baby'. It did fade eventually.)

Despite the birthmark and peeling skin, I thought my child was the most beautiful creation on earth. I held her hand and it felt soft as a rose petal and oh, so tiny! I admired her long straight legs. I held her dainty little feet and warmed them in my hand. I ran my finger along her well-defined, regal nose. I touched her little, perfectly shaped, soft pink lips. I stroked her dark hair and admired her neatly shaped ears. Her eyes opened and I saw the colours blue and brown mixed together to make a tone unique to her. And they were big and serious and they were looking at me. ME! Her mummy! I held her up close to my chest. The little head flopped about like a dislocated puppet against my shoulder. I put my hand over her tiny shoulders to steady her head and kissed my baby for the first time. I closed my eyes and whispered a little prayer to God, thanking Him for sending me this perfect little creature.

*

She was just twelve hours old when the crying started. It was the custom then, back in 1962, to keep the babies in the nursery at night so as to give the mums a good night's sleep. However, during the second night they wheeled Rachel into the ward at three a.m. and told me they couldn't get her to stop crying. They complained my daughter was disturbing all the other babies. It seemed, being her mother, I would automatically be endowed with some magical powers to deal with this distraught creature. I put her to a sore, empty breast. Held her, rocked her, whispered sweet nothings to her. Eventually she settled down.

Since the crying did not stop for longer than an hour or two at a time during the next few days, I begged the nurse to call a doctor to find out what was making her cry so. Eventually a doctor arrived. I explained to him that she was a rubella baby and could he tell me please if everything was all right with her. In front of me, he gave her a good examination, looked into her eyes, listened to her heart, checked out her spine and limbs, and finally told me he could find nothing physically wrong. I wanted to know why she was so fretful if there seemed to be no physical reason. He then told me the crying was due to her having an immature nervous system that would improve with time.

Lots of babies cry, I know. Rachel, however, cried almost constantly from twelve hours old until she was nine months. No doctor I took her to could find the cause or offer a remedy. The only thing that helped was a dummy and being cuddled and pushed in her pram. On her first outing, I remember as proud parents pushing her along the street to show our baby off to the world. However, our smiles changed to frowns when she screamed at the top of her lungs and would not let us enjoy this special time. That is until, in desperation, we called into the chemist and bought a dummy which I stuck into her mouth and – like incredible, beautiful magic – the crying stopped and our happiness returned.

*

During Rachel's first year, we moved into our own home. We had builders in to remove two walls to make the living area more spacious. The first clue we got that there might be something wrong with her, though it's only in hindsight, was that she slept right through the banging and drilling during the renovations. We all thought it was amusing to see her sleeping peacefully in her pram in the hallway while all hell broke loose around her.

The excitement of setting up our very first home distracted me from her crying for a while. Eventually the crying eased up once Rachel could crawl and get out of the pram. She even began repeating some simple words, delightfully, in my Scottish accent. I would hold her up in front of the mirror and point to her reflection, saying, 'Baby,' and she would repeat it. I would point to the birds hopping about in the garden and say, 'Bird,' and she would say, 'Bud' in my accent.

When she was about fifteen months she became ill. Great stringy projectiles of milk flew out of her mouth, accompanied by a loud, whooping sound. She had caught whooping cough, from somewhere or another.

Again, with the benefit of hindsight, it was only after that illness that she stopped repeating words; her chattering became warped and her squawking increased. Her hearing, which seemed normal up to that point, gradually decreased until finally it became obvious – not to me, as I had grown used to her way of communicating with me, but to observers.

Was it the whooping cough virus, or the rubella virus, or both, that did the damage? I suppose in the larger scheme of things it doesn't really matter. But at that time I still didn't know she had a hearing problem – it took an outside observer to point it out to me.

4

The diagnosis

One day when Rachel was almost two and I was about to give birth to my second child, we went to visit my sister. We were outside in the garden chatting over the fence with Pat's neighbour, Hilda, when Rachel ran past us and headed up towards the back garden. I called to her. She kept running. I called louder. Still she ignored me.

It was then that Hilda said, 'I don't think she can hear you, Margaret.'

After Hilda brought it to my attention, I made an appointment to see the paediatrician at Queen Charlotte's Hospital. (I had been told when she was born to bring her back when she was two if she was not talking.)

Again she was examined and given a cursory hearing test. The paediatrician stood behind her, close to her right ear, and clapped, softly at first, then gradually getting louder until there was a reaction and she turned her head to look up at him. He repeated it behind her left ear.

'There may be a loss,' he concluded. 'I'll give you a referral to an audiologist.'

I held on to the words 'may be a loss' and, again, put my head in the sand, refusing to consider this possibility.

In the meantime, on 9 November 1964, our second daughter, Judith, was born. At home. Upstairs. No fuss. No complications. Her birth was a joyful, happy distraction for a few months, and I had little time to worry about the possible outcome of the hearing test. It was nonetheless hovering in the background waiting to impart its news.

On the allotted date we went to the Heston Hearing Clinic. Heston is an outer suburb of London and a few suburbs away from our then home.

To my surprise, the staff greeted us with warmth and friendliness. This was a new and welcome experience for me. The audiologist was young and smiled brightly at me before crouching on his haunches to look into Rachel's eyes.

'Hello. What is your name?' he asked. He said this very slowly and I noticed he shaped his words well. It was our first lesson in lip-reading. She responded to this friendly man with a big smile. He pointed to her toy teddy, which she always carried with her. 'What is your teddy's name?'

She looked at him but just carried on smiling. I was about to talk for her but he held his hand up to me. I realised then he was ascertaining how much she could hear and understand.

'Shall we go into this room? We have a lot of toys for you to play with,' he continued slowly.

She looked at me. I couldn't help myself: I pointed at the door and nodded.

She nodded and the man said, 'OK, Rachel, let's go and see what we have in here for you.' He stood up, still keeping his eyes on Rachel, and walked towards the door. 'In here.'

We followed him inside. I was asked to sit on a low, small chair so that I was at Rachel's eye level. He sat on another small chair and opened a box. Inside was a drum, a tambourine and a few other noise-creating toys. The audiologist picked up the tambourine and began shaking it. All the time he was watching Rachel's reaction. She held out her hand for it and chattered in her own language. He seemed to understand her.

'You want to have a go too? Well, here you are.'

She took it and began shaking it close to her left ear.

'Nice sound?' he asked.

She just kept on shaking it. Then she turned to me and shook it in my ear.

I responded by nodding and saying, 'Nice sound,' just as he had done.

Then, while she was investigating the box of toys, he went behind her and began shaking the tambourine a few feet away. She did not respond. He came a little closer and shook it again. He repeated this until she finally turned round and put her hand out for it. In this way, he gradually built up a picture of her hearing capacity.

After a few more tests, he made a preliminary diagnosis. We went to his desk and talked while Rachel was happily playing with the toys.

'From this first test, it seems she has a moderate to severe hearing loss in both ears. We'll have to do more tests when she's a little older to get a more accurate result. In the meantime, we'll organise for Rachel to be fitted with two hearing aids. It's very important she begins to use them, as it'll bring her hearing up to reasonably workable level. What's happening now is that she's missing all the low pitches, so that male voices and most low sounds are lost to her. She also doesn't hear very high-pitched sounds such as "s" and "t" or medium sounds such as "m" and "n", or soft sounds, such as "p" and "b".'

My heart sank. 'You mean she can hear very little at all?' I could feel my eyes filling with tears.

He handed me a tissue and patted my hand. His kindness made me want to cry all the more. It was so good to know someone else understood how I was feeling right then.

'We'll do our very best to help your daughter. And you too. We have an excellent peripatetic teacher who will come to your home once a week. Jan will teach you how to communicate with Rachel. She'll also show you how to insert the aids properly.'

He got up and went to a drawer and pulled out some sheets of paper. He handed the first one to me. It showed a diagram of a harness in which to hold the aids on the outside of her clothes. 'It's better for the aids to be free of clothing – the sounds get distorted when fabric rubs against them,' he explained.

The second piece of paper was an invitation to come to a parents' evening that was being held in a couple of weeks' time, there at the clinic.

'Can you and your husband come? There's going to be a talk by an experienced teacher of the deaf. I think you'll find it useful.'

It was the first time the word 'deaf' had been used and it cut deep into my heart. Deaf! My child was officially deaf! I nodded, dumbly.

He reached across his desk and handed me another tissue. 'Rachel is a bright little girl, and we've caught her early. Two and a half is a good age to start her speech and listening training. A lot can be done for her.'

But for once I was silent and just looked at him and nodded.

A second appointment was made to have the impressions done for the earpieces. After that we went home.

Then I knew my life was changed for ever. I cried bitterly. My mother tried to comfort me with words that could never bring me solace. Rachel, who had been staring at me, went into the kitchen and brought me a tea towel and began wiping my eyes.

Mum laughed. 'This child is strong. She's going to get along well in life,' she declared with utter confidence.

Rachel stroked my face and chattered in her own language. She seemed to be telling me, 'My granny's right, Mummy. I'm going to be just fine.'

I held her close and hoped with all my heart they were right. But to me at that point, her future looked bleak and dark and hopeless.

5

Practicalities

Two weeks after the initial visit to the hearing clinic, David and I attended our first parents' meeting. The room was crowded. We sat near the back of the room. I thought, 'All these people have deaf children, like us.' It was no comfort.

I forget the speaker's name but remember vividly her vitality and passionate presentation of the subject matter as she walked to and fro in front of us. Only one thing she said that night has stayed in my mind because it was directed at David.

'Facial expressions are so important to a deaf child. Your expression, sir' – pointing at David – 'has not changed once for the past hour. Your child is going to have great difficulty understanding you.'

I looked at David and saw that he was staring into space. He neither reacted nor commented on this pronouncement, or showed that he had even understood what had been said to him. It was many years later before the question was raised that he might have Asperger's syndrome. Back then, I simply thought he was just a very shy sort of person who felt humiliated at being singled out like that. In any case, it set the pattern of his involvement – or rather non-involvement – in Rachel's early educational development.

The next thing to address was the hearing aids. After a month or so, we received her first aids. I bought the upholstery strips and sewed up her first harness. It had two separate pouches in which to hold the aids. Jan showed me how to insert the earpieces. I had to stand behind Rachel and gently but firmly push them into her ear. There was a lot of trouble getting it right, for she kept on pulling them out, or her ears became inflamed, itchy or tender. Eventually I decided, until she was older, just to have the one aid in her left ear. It was only years later, when she was able to speak, that I learned that the right aid made her right eye shake and cause visual problems. Back then, she simply refused to keep it in. And she would scream if I tried to insist.

The whistling from the aid when it became loose was always a problem; I was forever pushing the thing back into her ear. As she got older, she would do it herself, though sometimes she had to be reminded when the din drove us all mad.

As she grew older and could talk, she complained constantly that she didn't want to wear a hearing aid. I countered this just as constantly by telling her I hated wearing glasses but hated it more being unable to see properly, so I had to put up with them, just as she had to put up with having a hearing aid in her ear. That logic worked.

Another trick I developed to make her wear her aid was to simply refuse to talk to her unless it was in. That also worked, for she hated me to ignore her. Hated it!

The other problem was with wax build-up. This made her ear itch dreadfully and we were forever having it syringed and the wax removed from the earpiece.

Later on, the harness went when she was able to wear behind-the-ear aids. They hadn't been developed in the 60s or, if they had, they weren't available on the British or Australian health benefit schemes.

Cochlear implants only came into being towards the end of the century. By then Rachel had decided she would not take this risk as she had heard of a deaf person having a very bad psychological reaction because they could not adjust to having normal hearing. Up until now, at aged fifty, my daughter still resolutely refuses to consider this and puts up with itchy ears and poor-quality hearing devices. Or she simply refuses to wear them at all, most of the time, relying instead on her excellent lip-reading skills. (Rachel has commented on this in the second part of this book. Since writing our story, Rachel has decided to explore the possibility of having a cochlear implant.)

6

Other side effects

Another problem at the beginning was with Rachel's left eye. When she fixed her eyes on a given spot, the left one would slide to the outside edge of the socket. The eye specialist called it a 'divergent eye'. To remedy the problem, we had to put a plaster over the good eye so as to strengthen the lazy left eye muscle.

This, however, did not fix the problem. After a month or so, an appointment was made at the Children's Hospital in London, where she would have an operation to tighten the muscle. This involved a stay in hospital for a few days, which presented me with a dilemma. The hospital was too far away for me to travel to each day with baby Judy – what was I to do with her? Thankfully my mother and younger sister, Moira, came to the rescue and put us up in their cramped but very interesting and colourful hippie-style London flat.

I hugged Judy and started to say goodbye to her, saying I would see her after I had taken Rachel to the hospital. I was astonished at her reaction. Normally a very quiet, placid child, she screamed and clung on to me for dear life. Sixteen-year-old Moira took over and insisted I leave the baby with them and not worry, re-assuring me she would be just fine. In hindsight, could it perhaps have been the garish, hippie decorations that freaked out this totally left-brain-oriented child who would later grow up to be a teacher of mathematics and a no-nonsense sort of a girl?

The eye operation helped a little. Nevertheless, throughout Rachel's childhood I would have to remind her to bring her eye 'back' whenever I saw it drifting outwards. It didn't seem to affect her sight, which, thankfully was perfect.

As I type this, a vision of another rubella child popped into my head. The child was blind and deaf. When I first saw her, she was in the grounds of the Heston Clinic. She was trying to play but her body was folded almost in half, her hands stretched out in front of her, trying to orientate herself towards the dim sounds she could hear around her. Any self-pity I had for my own daughter's disability fell into a more reasonable perspective at that moment and I silently thanked God for our good fortune.

That is not to say that Rachel got away with just her hearing being damaged by the rubella virus. Other problems presented themselves as time went on.

One such side effect I learned from her first teacher at the Opportunity for the Deaf (OD) Unit was the size of her hands. They are tiny. As are her feet and toes. I remember Miss Large saying when she first met Rachel and saw her hands, 'Oh yes, she has stunted hands and feet. It's the rubella – it stunts their growth. She won't reach her natural height.' She said this so casually and was obviously totally unaware of, or perhaps simply uninterested in, my sensitive feelings. I had these horrible visions of my daughter being a small, distorted dwarf when she grew up. I am happy to say that, apart from her tiny hands and feet, she finally reached a reasonable height – at least one inch taller than my 5' 2" but way shorter than her (comparatively) strapping 5' 6" and 5' 7" three younger sisters.

When she was eight or so, Rachel began complaining about sore wrists. I took her to the doctor and he diagnosed arthritis. She was put on a course of aspirin which helped ease the swelling and pain. Unfortunately she couldn't stay on aspirin indefinitely for I feared liver damage. I took her to an acupuncturist but stopped this treatment after I learned that it worked by killing the nerves of the affected joint. I didn't want her to have numb wrists. We tried instead certain diets – not to much effect. She still gets attacks of arthritis and both her wrists are distorted with the disease. Sometimes she cannot use her hands. Rachel bears these discomforts bravely and philosophically.

*

A pattern throughout her childhood was that Rachel hated walking, running, or doing sport. The only exercise she enjoyed was swimming. I only have one memory of her ever enjoying physical activity. She must have been close to three at the time. We were visiting sister Pat and decided to take the two cousins (two months apart in age) to their local park. In this park was a giant slippery slide. Rachel ran towards it, quickly climbed up the steps, turned and beckoned her more hesitant cousin to follow. Not waiting for Hilary, my girl jumped onto the shining chute, let go and, laughing excitedly, zipped down and straight into my waiting arms. I remember feeling secretly proud of my fearless daughter as her more cautious cousin trailed after her that day.

That was a rare moment, though. As she grew older, her reluctance to walk, run or expend energy of any kind slowly increased.

Because she couldn't communicate, I wondered if there was something physically wrong with her legs, hips or spine that made physical exertion such a problem for her. I had her checked out. Nothing was found to be wrong. (It is only now that Rachel has told me that her feet and legs ached when she walked.)

I wonder why she was always so tired as a child and unwilling to do anything that put any strain on her body? It is easy to blame the rubella – I blame everything negative on the viral damage – but what if it was nothing more than her nature and she would have been like it anyway, virus or no virus?

In her mid 20s Rachel was diagnosed as having a schizo-affective disorder. Later still, she developed glandular fever and a malfunctioning thyroid. Recently she has discovered her heart had moved to the right side. For a while, diabetes was diagnosed but seemingly it cleared up after the thyroid operation. She is currently having her eyesight checked as she has developed 'a pale patch' in her left eye (see Appendix).

Not one of the many medical professionals we consulted pinpointed these problems as being the result of rubella damage. However, when neither I, nor any of my other daughters, had any of these ailments, how can I not put it all down to rubella?

Another question has formulated in my mind as I write this in 2012. Why did the medical profession not come to this conclusion? Is it because so little was known about rubella damage? In the 1960s it was virtually impossible for parents to find out about all the possible affects. I wonder if the medical authorities were similarly ignorant back then? Today I can click onto the internet and find out almost everything about rubella.

7

Early training

Things started happening quickly after the initial diagnosis at the Heston Hearing Clinic. Once it was discovered that Rachel had a serious hearing loss, it was all systems go to get her rehabilitated.

The first thing to happen was a visit from the peripatetic teacher. Jan arrived in my home, brisk, professional and very sophisticated to my young and untrained eyes. She was tall, blonde, slim, about 36ish, American and married to a doctor. They had five children of their own; the youngest, like Rachel, was a rubella child, quite deaf but 'doing swell'.

Jan got to work straight away with my training. The first thing I learned was that we must always face the child when we speak to them. Get down to their level, eye to eye, so they can see your mouth and facial expressions clearly. 'In this manner, they learn more quickly,' she explained.

She also explained that because Rachel was on the borderline between being profoundly deaf and partially hearing, she would be trained as a partially hearing child. 'There's a big difference,' Jan said. There would be no sign language involved. Rachel would learn to lip-read and make the most use of her available hearing. I would train her (with Jan's help) to speak as clearly as possible.

'When Rachel is a little older, she'll start at the Opportunity for the Deaf Unit attached to the Heston Public School, where she'll receive intensive speech training,' she explained. 'Eventually she,ll be integrated into the hearing classes. We don't ever use the word "normal". We say, "hearing school situation",' she added.

In the meantime, Jan would arrange for Rachel to attend the local kindergarten, three mornings a week, until she was old enough to go to school.

At the end of the first hour with me, Jan left in an efficient breeze. Her parting words were not so comforting. 'It's harder for you, honey – your first child being handicapped. My boy has his siblings to help and encourage him. But we'll do the very best we can for your darling little girl. So long. I'll be seeing you same time next Tuesday.'

*

Jan came along faithfully every Tuesday morning and brought games and toys and teaching aids to help me with Rachel's training. She was a great inspiration to me and I found myself devising my own games to help my daughter to understand words that we naturally use simply because we are exposed to them all the time. One of the most difficult concepts to get over to hearing people is that, if you are born deaf and only hear gurgling sounds when people speak, how on earth can you, a deaf person, copy language? It simply is not possible. Until deaf people are taught each and every word, step by step and repeated many times, they will never be able to speak properly, or even understand the meaning of words.

Once I understood this, I went to work to bring language to my child as fast as I possibly could. And Rachel was a very willing learner. She naturally loved words, books, songs and letters. It was a joy to play these learning games with her. I purchased a book and word pack set called *Teach Your Baby to Read*. I bought a pack of snap cards, and every night before going to sleep we would play our reading game. I chose three written words from the *Teach Your Baby to Read* word pack, and also three pictures of the same subject. I would then hold up, say, a picture of a banana, then the word banana and point to them both. Banana for the word, then banana for the picture and say the word 'banana' and ask her to repeat the word back to me. If she couldn't get the 'n' sound, I put her hand to my throat so she could feel the vibrations of the 'n' sound. Then put my hand to her throat and ask her to say the word 'banana', which she did, putting her own hand on her throat and feeling the vibration of the 'n' sound as well.

To help her learn to use her hearing, I would then ask her to point to the word I was saying while I covered my mouth. And she would listen very carefully and pick up the picture of the sound-word I was saying. And we would work through the other words and pictures and pronunciations until she had learned them all thoroughly.

This went on for the next few months. Then of course, this naturally followed in our everyday life. I would point to a chair and say 'chair' and ask her to tell me what it was. Then I would cover my mouth and again repeat the word, chair, table, sock, shoe and so on – whatever it was we were learning that day.

Then I devised a game of abstract words, such as 'on', 'under', 'up', 'down' and so on. At first I'd point to each place so that she understood where I wanted her to put things, then cover my mouth and say, 'Put the shoe under the chair.' Then I would ask her to put the shoe on the chair. She would listen carefully then do it. I of course gave her lots of applause and smiles and encouragement when she got it right.

In this way, Rachel learned how to speak, read and understand concepts that hearing people take for granted, day in and day out.

*

When she was three, she started at the Opportunity for the Deaf Unit attached to the Heston Public School. Because of her willingness to learn from my teaching, she was able to read, identify and say thirty words at a time when other hearing-impaired infants were still struggling to make sense of even the simplest of concepts and words.

She was a bright, outgoing, friendly and curious child, always wanting to learn new things. It was easy to help her.

*

Another very valuable learning tool that I was introduced to was the idea of the weekend news diary. Rachel came home from school with a blank exercise book with a note saying, 'Would you please make a picture of something that happened over the weekend so that the children can discuss it at school on Monday mornings.'

This became a regular Sunday evening exercise. We chose some event that had happened over the weekend and at first I drew little stick figures to go with the words. This progressed very quickly to actual drawings of things to make it more interesting and intelligible for Rachel.

Before she left that school, we had filled up a great many of those wretched diaries. Only one has survived. It is now kept in a safe place for posterity. As a result of this drawing, Rachel in later years took up painting and still enjoys painting to this day. She also had her artwork exhibited a few years ago.

*

And so Rachel's education progressed. She still could not put whole, simple sentences together until she was seven or eight-years old. Her frustration at not being able to express her wants was terrible and we all had to endure many screaming tantrums through the years until her speech improved to a level where she could reason and talk about her needs in a sensible and quiet, civilised manner.

This idea of insisting upon making children with a partial hearing loss learn to use their residual hearing by using lip-reading and intensive speech training was only introduced in Britain (I believe) in the early 1960s. Before that, all children with a hearing impairment went into a special school for the deaf and learned to communicate with sign language. These children never learned to use their voice, or did so with little success. This set them apart, thus isolating them from normal society, hence the new philosophy behind the push to train those children with a partial loss to communicate like the hearing population. The idea was to integrate them into ordinary society.

Did it work out? I asked Rachel this question. Her answer is in part two of this book.

8

Battle of wills

Jan came regularly every Tuesday for many weeks. She helped me have Rachel enrolled in the local kindergarten, or nursery to give it its British name. Because of Rachel's disability, the fee was funded by the government. I was later to discover she would obtain many benefits to assist her in her life. This was the first.

The nursery school was at the end of our street and across a busy road, about a mile away. On the way there, Rachel walked quickly beside Judy's pram. She looked forward to going and playing with the children, for she was a gregarious, outgoing little girl and loved company. She waved me goodbye happily and not once did she cry when I left. After lunch, I returned to pick her up.

It was at this stage that I experienced my greatest trouble with her. She seemed happy to leave the nursery, waving goodbye to everyone and setting off across the busy road to start on the walk to our house. Once out of sight of the nursery and at the stretch of road leading to our house, she stopped walking. Simply refused to take another step! When I insisted, she screamed and sat down on the pavement. I would haul her up again and pull her along while pushing the pram with my other hand, she screaming blue murder and me grim-faced and equally determined not to give in to her. Yes, I know I could have put her in the pram with Judy, but why should I? She was well able to walk to the nursery; it was the same distance back again. OK, I can hear you saying, 'She could have been feeling tired after her morning at the nursery. Couldn't you have relented and squashed her into the pram, for goodness sake?'

Yes, I could have. Had I been the mature woman I am now, of course I would have, but I was still immature. I myself hadn't yet learned to give way to someone else's will. I was a stubborn, self-willed person and besides I was the boss and she had to bend to my will, not force me to bend to hers. That is how it was with us. And it has caused us many a mighty battle, especially difficult because there was no way I could reason or bribe her into doing things my way or at least get her to agree to meet me halfway. It was her way or it would be hell on earth.

Both of us having a stubborn, unbending nature made bringing her up very difficult for both of us and, unfortunately, for the rest of the family, who had to witness our constant battles of wills. David would take off to the bathroom, Judy would slink off to the bedroom and baby Holly sneaked out to the garden to play with the dog when one of the storms hit. Rachel always won because she had learned that if she screamed long enough I would give in, give her what she wanted and cuddle her into the bargain.

These tantrums lasted throughout her childhood. One in particular sticks out in my mind. Rachel would have been twelve or thirteen at the time. We had gone out for a family trip to Manly by ferry. We had, as usual, a pleasant day. It was on the way home when we decided to walk from Circular Quay and up George Street, intending to catch the train from Town Hall. I suppose Rachel must have been feeling overtired. But we all were. Even six-year-old Holly trotted along quietly without complaining. Then, halfway along George Street, Rachel sat down in a doorway and refused to walk any further. Of course we got annoyed with her and insisted she got up right away. She simply refused! What could we do? There was nothing for it but to flop down beside her and wait until she was ready to walk again.

*

So, what was the reason for these emotional meltdowns – this inability to keep control of her emotions? Just not being able to communicate with us? Did other deaf children behave like this? Or was this peculiar to Rachel? Was it possible that her nervous system was damaged, along with her hearing, by the rubella virus?

I asked Rachel if she would like to write a few words. Her spontaneous and startlingly impressive reply, included in the second half of this book, was quickly forthcoming.

9

Early schooling

Once the kindergarten experiment was over, Jan talked to me about Rachel's future. 'We're not sure whether Rachel's hearing loss is severe enough for her to be enrolled in the Heston Hearing Impaired Unit. She's borderline, Margaret. The idea is to integrate the children into the hearing world if possible, and as soon as is possible. She's doing swell with your help. How do you feel about this?'

The decision was not really difficult to make because I knew Rachel would get intensive speech training and an opportunity to build up reading skills in a sheltered, caring situation. After a moment's hesitation, I said, 'I want the best help possible, Jan. I feel it would be better for her to get at least two years of intensive speech training before going into a public school. Right now she can't even put two words together, can she?

Jan looked at me as if considering my opinion carefully. I can still see her standing before me, deciding on my daughter's future. I knew she would have preferred me to choose the hearing environment but she did not try to push me to make that decision.

She closed her briefcase and began walking towards the front door. 'That's settled then, Margaret. I'll get the ball rolling and be in touch soon. This will be our last meeting today. I'll be seeing Rachel at Heston from now on.' And with that, my lifeline and inspiration left me to my own devices.

I kept up the reading at night and the learning of as many new words as Rachel was willing to soak up.

*

Within a couple of months, we had the date set for Rachel's first day. She would be picked up by a taxi service every morning and brought back after school. That was to be her way of getting to and from school for the next few years.

There was great excitement on her first day when she left home all by herself. I can still see her happy, smiling face peering out of the back window as the car whisked her away on her great new adventure. Rachel loves all things new. She is never happier than when a new situation presents itself and she has to experience it thoroughly. This is her elixir of life. She was just three and a half years old when she began this new, exciting journey.

*

As the weeks turned to months her scribble-talk changed. Instead of a constant babble of meaningless sounds, I could detect some English phrases.

After a year's intensive speech training, she could string together very simple sentences. She was always talking about 'Mi La' – Miss Large, her teacher. I eventually got tired of hearing about 'Mi La' and began teaching her how to say Miss Large. For the 'm' sound I put her hand on my throat so she could feel the 'm' vibration, then put both her hands on her throat. Eventually she got the humming sound, which pleased us both enormously. The same with 's' – 'Missss, Rachel'. I would hold her hand up to my mouth so that she could feel the air against her hand as I made the 's' sound and she copied me. After a few tries we had 'Miss Laaje'.

As time went on I would do the same with 't', 'k', 'p', sounds. In this way, her speech training progressed smoothly for the next three years or so at the hearing unit.

One last problem I will mention here is that her voice – like most deaf children – was nasal. She spoke without using the lower register and it sounded tinny and artificial. I again put my hand on my throat when I talked so that she could feel the vibrations lower down. Then I would make her repeat the words, ensuring her throat hummed and vibrated.

After a while, whenever she forgot, I would just put my hand straight out then press my palm downwards towards the floor and she understood and lowered the pitch to a normal level.

*

Once Rachel went off to school, my life settled into a quiet routine. I had time to enjoy my other baby, Judy. Judy was very different from Rachel. I spent many a peaceful hour watching her play quietly by herself. Judy loved to investigate everything. She would pick up an object, anything at all, turn it around in her hands, tap, twist, taste, shake. When it had been thoroughly examined, it was unceremoniously discarded in favour of something new. Every now and then, she would come to me and hold her arms up for a cuddle. She loved nothing more than to be cuddled, and I was more than willing to cuddle this peaceful child. Sometimes she brought a book to me, climbed onto my lap and listened quietly as I read it to her. She rarely asked questions or commented on the story; she simply listened and absorbed. She seldom cried. She hardly ever smiled. She was just there, calm and placid and no trouble at all.

When Judy turned three, I took her to the local playgroup centre, then – all too soon – it was time for her to go to school. I hated leaving Judy at school. I missed her quiet companionship.

10

Our new life in Australia

Two months after Judy began school, our lives changed completely; we had been accepted by the Australian government as residents of their country. On a cold, wet day in November 1969, we left our native land, family and friends and set sail. After six unforgettable weeks on board ship, we arrived at Sydney Harbour.

I fell in love with Sydney at first sight. I adored the vast deep blue empty sky, the lights twinkling in houses that nestled amongst sweet-scented trees, the white-hot sun and canopied shops, the quaint old trains they called red rattlers, with windows you could open and, amazingly, no closed doors in the entrances! Top of the list were, of course, the fabulous white sandy beaches and sparkling blue sea with enormous white-tipped rolling waves.

We sailed away from a bleak, black and white, unfriendly, overcrowded country, and sailed into a technicoloured wonderland. Most pleasing to me were the friendly Australians who smiled at us and said 'G'day' when we passed them in the street, and shop assistants who, back then, had the time for a quick chat and actually eyeballed their customers when exchanging goods for cash.

There were many new words for Rachel (and all of us) to learn. The very first being 'huntsmen', 'bindies', 'mozzies', 'reserves' (for parks). We were 'good' not 'well' when asked how we were. More came as time went on.

They must have been confusing to seven-year-old Rachel, whose knowledge of English was just beginning to make sense. To add to her confusion was the change in dialect. How difficult must this have been for her; undoubtedly it was the cause of her increased temper tantrums and screaming fits.

David and Judy seemed to take these changes in their stride, but I suffered from acute loneliness. Suddenly we were such a small family; just the four of us. One deaf child who couldn't speak; one quiet, placid child, content simply to be hugged; and one husband who lived in his own world, who smiled and chatted to himself when he thought I wasn't looking but presented a face of stone across the dining table whenever I talked longingly about the family I'd so cheerfully waved goodbye to a year or so before.

The remedy, I thought, was another child, or many more children to increase our own family – bring more life and chattering into our unit.

Holly was that child. She arrived on 13 August 1971; my fearless, courageous daughter (who would later become a world kickboxing champion,) bringing life and energy into my life and joy into my heart.

11

Penshurst Opportunity for the Deaf Unit

Rachel's education continued in the hearing-impaired Opportunity for the Deaf (OD) Unit attached to the public school in Penshurst, a suburb in Sydney's west. We were living in Bankstown, which was about fifteen kilometres further west, therefore requiring the taxi service to convey her to and from school. Because of the change in culture, language and environment, I did not consider starting her at the local primary school along with Judy. When she had settled into her new environment she would gradually integrate in stages into the hearing classes. This seemed the sensible and most practical course to take.

*

My mother always said to us when we were children, 'Comparisons are odious.' Therefore I write this chapter with some trepidation for I don't want to appear like some ignoramus making derogatory statements about something about which I know nothing – as was the case when I was a child. My comparisons are based on my own personal experience, therefore valid. So, please, my Australian friends, do not take umbrage at what I am about to write next.

The quality of the hearing-impaired education facilities in London in the 1960s and those the teachers and students in the Penshurst OD Unit in Sydney had to contend with was like going from a millionaire's home to that of a pauper. Our children here in Australia missed a great deal of learning, both in speech development and reading and writing because of the third-world facilities in their classrooms.

The OD unit in London, where Rachel attended until the age of seven, was well equipped to produce the best possible hearing quality in the classroom. The floors and walls were carpeted to absorb as much external noise as possible. There was a loop system in each of the classrooms so that each child's aid picked up the best individual sound quality as the teacher spoke. The teaching materials were rich and abundant. The children flourished under the expert teaching methods and, by the time we left to come to Australia, Rachel had had a well-rounded education. Her reading and writing skills almost equalled the children in the hearing classes. At times the hearing-impaired children integrated with the hearing ones in such things as art, drama, music and sport.

Unfortunately, this was not the case when we came to live in Australia. The hearing-impaired classes had no carpeting or special teaching equipment. The children had poor speech development, and reading skills were poor in comparison with the British equivalent. I am not saying this in a derogatory way. The teachers themselves were just as dedicated and skilful as their British peers, but the equipment was poor and the funding totally inadequate. The needs of the children obviously were not well understood at that time. I'm talking about 1969/1970 when the Liberal government was in power.

It was not until the Labor prime minister, Gough Whitlam, arrived and money was made available for education, that the OD unit saw improvements. Rachel was nine by then and her academic level had virtually stagnated. Her behaviour, as well as that of the other children, was poor. She came home constantly with bruises on her legs and arms which had resulted from rough play and fighting with her schoolmates. Since their speech was so poor, these children communicated physically. I heard tales of them jumping on desks, throwing things about the rooms and generally mucking up, and also fighting with the hearing children in the playground.

However, despite the poor facilities, Rachel did progress academically. When she was eleven, they decided to try integrating her in the hearing class for some of the time.

One day the principal of the OD unit called me in to school to report on Rachel's performance during integration. I was surprised when she told me quite bluntly that Rachel was not doing well in the integrated classroom situation. Of course I wanted to know why she had come to this conclusion.

She told me, 'Rachel is a child who only works when she's being constantly supervised. When she's left alone to do things by herself, she stops working and waits until she gets attention. She will never integrate into the hearing world.'

Was she right? At that stage I was completely unwilling to accept this analysis of my child's character. Rather I felt it was as a result of the poor teaching methods that had been used to educate the children in the OD unit. It had lacked direction and stimulation for a bright child such as Rachel. She had simply never been encouraged to use her initiative.

I took her out of the OD unit and put her into the local public school, where I felt sure she would prove them wrong and swim her way through school, through her life.

The local school, Bankstown West Public School, welcomed Rachel with all the good-hearted mateship for which Australians are famous. The school captain, Christine Finch, took her under her wing. Everyone did their best to help this strange girl with the hearing aid, bright smile and a string of barely coherent sentences as her entertainment value. She loved all the attention. Loved being thought special and she flourished. She walked to school with Judy, who was one class down. They came home together. They became normal schoolmates for the first time. This is not to say they became buddies. They were never that. The communication difficulties between them were still there. They fought sometimes. Sometimes they played together when there was some physical action involved, such as hide and seek, or playing on the swings, or swimming. Sometimes they played board games, such as Ludo and Snakes and Ladders, or card games. However, they never could sit together and chat like normal sisters. It grew worse as they grew older. And there was simply nothing I could do to help them. There was no sign language allowed. Judy couldn't understand what Rachel was saying and vice versa. Holly, being seven years younger than Judy, could not then participate in these activities. (Holly was later to learn sign language and briefly become an interpreter in a school situation.)

Did Rachel miss her deaf friends? I don't recall now her ever visiting them again. I did not encourage her to keep in touch with them, I admit. I wanted her to integrate into the hearing world. I wanted her to find new friends, ordinary girls.

When she turned twelve, she started high school. The girls from Bankstown West continued on to Bankstown Girls High. She made some new friends there and her life at school progressed satisfactorily. Her lip-reading skills developed well, her speech improved and she passed all her exams with reasonable marks, including obtaining the School Leaving Certificate in Year 10. I was content with her progress. I assumed her education would continue into Year 12 and she would receive the High School Certificate. But things changed dramatically just after she started Year 11.

12

New beginnings

Rachel had only been in Year 11 for about two months when Judy came to me one day and said, 'Mum, something's wrong with Rachel. She's up at Dad's house and she's acting strangely.' (By this time our marriage had broken down and we lived two streets apart.)

I will never forget the sight that met me as I walked into the house. Rachel was standing with her back to the wall, both arms spread apart, her palms pressed firmly against the wall as if to support herself and keep from collapsing to the floor. Her face was flushed and her eyes bright and staring straight ahead. She seemed unaware of us.

Judy brought an empty bottle of sea sickness tablets from the kitchen.

'Oh, my God, Rachel! What's happened to you?' I screamed, totally off of my head with worry.

She couldn't talk. I got her to drink warm, salty water and made her vomit by sticking my fingers down her throat until she retched and threw up.

We somehow managed to half-carry, half-drag her into the car and back to our townhouse and upstairs to bed. I went into damage control mode, quickly deciding it was as a result of her being in Year 11, where the work was a lot harder and she just wasn't coping with it. I asked her if that was the problem. She nodded. I left her to sleep it off.

Instead of taking Rachel to a doctor and getting this attempt at suicide investigated, I decided it was all because the school work was simply too difficult for a hearing-impaired person to grasp and immediately took her out of high school. I had her enrolled in a business college, where she learned about office work and acquiring typing skills.

The change in environment seemed to have a positive effect on Rachel for there were no further signs of the emotional breakdown she had experienced a few months before. I felt convinced it had all been due to the school work being too much for her and put it out of my mind; after all, my own remedy had worked. By the end of the year she had completed the course and arrived home proudly displaying her business certificate. Armed with this qualification, we went to an employment agency that dealt with people with disabilities. They gave her a typing test that she passed with a reasonable speed. Again she got a certificate to show to future employers.

Then we looked for work. We saw an advertisement placed in the papers by Telecom in the Sydney CBD for data entry operators with typing skills. (No data entry experience necessary, as training would be given to the successful applicants, the ad said, helpfully.) She applied and was successful.

*

Rachel was employed by Telecom for many years. She met some new friends, hearing as well as deaf, and her life took off. She learned to drive and bought her first car. She travelled overseas three times, took up oil painting, had a nice boyfriend, and had plenty of friends.

She joined the Deaf Club in Sydney and was overjoyed to meet up with her former school friends from the OD Unit in Penshurst. They were all now using sign language to communicate with one another. Rachel quickly decided to learn how to do this.

After a while she brought her friends home and with dismay I watched them signing. They used a mixture of language and signing, both unintelligible to me. For the first time I felt excluded from my daughter and her friends.

Rachel brought a large book of Auslan sign language for me to learn. I couldn't do it. I couldn't see the point of learning to sign when we had spent all of our lives desperately trying to bring language to our partially hearing children. Now it seemed they all preferred to communicate together with sign language. Of course I can understand why. The question is, why were they put through all that trauma of learning to speak in the first place? Why were all of us put through it – the children, our families? It seemed a pointless exercise to me. But was it in the long run, I wonder. Have the children benefited or not? Rachel's comments are set out in the second part of this book.

In the meantime, I will finish this first stage of Rachel's life by introducing the man who played a major part in her new life. His name is Daniel Corte.

13

Danny

Rachel had known Danny for quite some time before I finally met him. He was part of her deaf group of friends. She liked him. 'He makes me laugh,' she said. She brought him to meet me.

He was a tall, handsome man, in his mid-twenties. He sat beside Rachel and looked at me benignly, expectantly.

I realised he was waiting for me to chat to him. So I said, 'Hello, Danny. How are you?'

He nodded and raised his thumb in the Auslan sign for 'Good'.

'He can't speak, Mum. He can't read or write.'

'So how do I talk to him, Rachel?' I said, smiling but in quiet desperation, for I could tell by the way they looked at each other that this was going to be more than a passing fancy. This man could become my future son-in-law.

'You have to learn sign language so you can talk to him,' she said simply.

'I'll try, but right now do you think you can you interpret for me? Ask Danny what he does.' (The eternal parental question.)

She made rapid finger movements and exaggerated facial expressions. He returned them, intriguingly slicing his hand across his throat, pulling an imaginary rope up and twisting his neck grotesquely to the side, sticking his tongue out and crossing his eyes. At the end of this performance, he sat forward and looked at me again in his gentle, kindly way.

'He wrings chickens' necks.'

'Oh!'

He tapped Rachel and held up all of his fingers, then turned down two and nodded vigorously.

'He says he's been doing it for eight years.'

'Well!' I was myself dumbfounded. The mere thought of this gentle guy wringing thousands of chickens' necks was simply mind-boggling.

He leaned forward, rubbed his fingers together and again raised his thumb in the 'good' sign, accompanied by the nodding.

I was getting it. 'Ah, good money, huh!' I said, smiling and nodding vigorously in return.

Then he stood up and began revving up an imaginary motorbike, gave the thumbs up and nodded again.

'You've got a motorbike?'

Again he answered with the thumbs up and fast nods. He then turned an imaginary car wheel, and made a gesture that looked as if he was saying he loved something very much and it cost him a lot of money. He pushed two imaginary doors closed and turned a key.'

Rachel laughed. 'He's telling you about his pride and joy. He's got a big Kingston in his garage. He doesn't use it because he's keeping it special.'

'Oh, I see! Does he like cakes, Rachel?' I suddenly wanted to spoil this young man rotten.

I was to discover pretty soon that he had been fostered as a baby. A woman called Dawn had brought him up. He was profoundly deaf and had spent his entire schooling at North Rocks School for the Deaf and Blind. He had never been taught to speak. When he did try to say some words they were totally distorted, so he preferred to be mute. His surname was Corte. Dawn told us his father was Italian, but she had never met him. She said she didn't know anything about his real mother, or where she was.

It was only later when Rachel became pregnant that Dawn revealed the truth about his mother. She told Rachel Danny's mother was also deaf, and that he had some sisters and brothers. She either didn't know or refused to tell Danny where his real mother was living.

I had a serious talk with Rachel when she became pregnant. I asked her whether she was willing to risk having a child that might inherit Danny's genetic deafness.

She looked seriously at me for a moment, and then she said, 'It's a risk I'm going to take, Mum. Danny and I want to get married.'

*

And here I will leave Rachel's story. I have concentrated on my experiences with bringing up a severely deaf child. I have ended where my work with her finished and she had been successfully launched into her adult life.

Was it all worth it?

A few weeks ago I visited Rachel and watched her chatting with her eight-year-old daughter. The child was sitting crossed legged on the chair opposite Rachel telling her mother something or another. Back and forward the dialogue went. No trouble. No effort. A warm glow filled my being seeing them chatting together as Rachel and I never could (at that age).

Yes. For me it was worth every bit of effort, every storm, confusion and tantrum. This is my reward.

Now I am honoured and privileged to bring to you Rachel's experiences as a young deaf girl as seen from her own perspective.

Part two

Rachel's Story

Being deaf

For me personally, I feel that being able to speak has a lot of advantages over sign language in helping me to integrate within the hearing world but most of my partial-hearing friends argue the fact that we are born deaf and it is the right of deaf people to use sign language as their natural method of communication.

I have been partially deaf myself from birth, but in my forties my hearing deteriorated to profound hearing loss. I can still hear very well with stronger hearing aids. The audiologist once remarked that he was astounded at how well I can listen to sounds. But being deaf is a daily struggle – it has been all my life – to keep listening to the spoken language to get it right, as I tend to miss a few words in a sentence and lots of misunderstanding lies there. It's pretty frustrating to have to live with that. That is the difficulty of being deaf: not being able to enjoy the free-flowing comprehension of the conversations that hearing people take for granted.

As a child, I had no inkling that I was different nor was I aware that I had a hearing problem till I was seven years old. I remember that my relationship with my mother was very frustrating because I couldn't understand why she could not understand me when I tried to tell her things. My father would nod at everything I said. My sister Judy was a very quiet child, said very little, but we played normal stuff without any misunderstanding. Holly was a baby. I was nine when she was born. There was not much talking between us.

I don't really know why I cried a lot as child. It could be that my nervous system wasn't fully developed as a result of the rubella, but I remember the feelings were so sharp and intense, the environment around me was highly very sensitive to my soul, and this would trigger crying bouts and tantrums. Being very sensitive, like my mother, I could feel all emotions around people; I could sense what others were thinking. This really caused confusion in my psyche, and not being able to explain my feelings made me feel very frightened. I couldn't tell my mother this because I didn't know how to tell her. That's why I had terrible tantrums with my mother. I learned to keep my feelings to myself as I grew up.

There's one example I can remember when we were on the ship. We were on the bottom deck, close to the engine of the ship; I could hear the engine humming. For years after that I could hear the engine humming when I was asleep or waking up. That feeling faded over the years. Why did the ship noise linger? I could never understand it. Still don't.

I was seven years old when I first discovered that I was deaf. One day my parents took me and my sister to the beach. Upon returning from the beach, my neighbour at the flat at Lakemba where we used to live when we moved here from England asked me what I had done that day,

I replied, 'I went to the beach.' I must have said, 'I went to beeee.' She asked what I had said and I told her again, 'I went to the beach,' but she could not understand me so I made my arms swim around, like I was swimming, then she understood. That was when realisation hit me. I was questioning myself, wondering why she didn't understand me and why I had to repeat myself to make myself understood to some people. Then I noticed my hearing aid and realised that my family or others were not wearing one as well.

I asked, 'Why, Mum, I wear this?'

She said, 'Rachel, you're deaf. You can't hear.'

I remember feeling shocked. Realising that people were not going to understand me really upset me greatly. I knew then that what my mother had been doing to teach me to speak properly was so important. But after that realisation, I became very self-conscious and shy when I spoke to people. It was a very uncomfortable feeling. And of course,

I couldn't tell my mum what had happened with that incident with the neighbour because I didn't know how to explain it to her as I still couldn't get my sentences right. So I kept it to myself, feeling rather lonely with this new knowledge.

When I attended Penshurst Primary School with the OD Unit, I observed a lot about my deafness and my deaf peers. As my mother said, I was getting the right training of my speech but lacked what I had in the English school. It was a bare classroom. Just tables and chairs and blackboard. We were taught to lip-read and also to then cover our mouth and try to hear sounds without lip-reading. And we were trained to listen for different background sounds. Listening to music played an important part as well. Eventually they got a new machine, like a tape recorder, for us to learn to hear our voices and learn to speak properly. I was a very willing learner and loved hearing my voice on that machine; it really helped me to speak clearly. It was further two years before I could make myself understood.

Another thing I had to deal with was bullying by an older deaf girl; she would bully each of us each week. One day my friend cried when it was her turn to be bullied.

When I went home that day I asked my mother, 'Why do we cry?'

Mum replied the best she could, telling me it's because our feelings are hurt. I pondered this new concept for a while. I was surprise by 'feelings'. I was completely unaware that others felt things, not just me. This was my first understanding of emotions. I was about eight or nine years old. This is when I first stood up to this bullying girl, and of course, I copped a lot from her, hence the bruises on my legs! But I gained respect from other deaf children, who sought my protection.

One of my early memories at that school was when I asked my teacher for a felt pen. My teacher didn't understand what I wanted so she asked me to write it on the blackboard. I wrote, 'felt pen' and still she didn't understand what it was. Then she asked me to find one in the cupboard where all the stationery was placed. I took out the felt pen box and showed it to her, and then she said, 'Oh, you mean texta.'

She saw that I was confused and wrote 'texta' on the blackboard and explained to me the right word to use. She had never heard of felt pens before. But I was still confused. I didn't understand why there were two names for them. I didn't understand the difference between the English and Australian languages. I was seven years old at the time. I told my mother about felt pens and textas. I asked her why there were two names. I wanted an answer, but of course she didn't understand my speech, and it wasn't till later years, when I could speak properly, that I asked her the question again.

It all boils down the fact that I knew things I wanted to discuss with my mother, but could never do; I would give my screaming tantrums to her, and at times cried constantly in my sleep. I could never talk to my sisters, Judy and Holly, or my dad because they were so quiet and uncommunicative, but I could play games with them and took great joy in that.

Another confusing matter in the classroom was that the older deaf boys would draw the swastika on the blackboard and salute 'Hitler' and would make us to do the same. I had no idea who Hitler was but the boys would get caned for it. Later in my teen years, I did a history subject on Hitler and World War II, and then I understood. It was funny that the teachers in primary school didn't want to talk about Hitler; it was forbidden to talk about him. After all, it was the early 70s. I think one of the deaf boys had a German family background and made an issue out of it. I faintly remember that his father was a German; he boasted about it. I really thought what a strange school that was, so different from its British counterpart.

I have little memory of my British school, except my teacher, Miss Large, and my two best friends, Helen Palmer and Catherine.

I remember the day my mother told me that we were flying to Australia. We were sitting on the porch when a plane flew overhead and my mother pointed to it and said to me, 'We're going on one of those to Australia.'

Miss Large had shown us a picture of a kangaroo, telling everyone that I would be seeing one, and of course I was so excited and felt special to be seeing one. I thought, what a big exciting adventure. But we went on a ship instead. It was because my mother was allergic to the smallpox shot that she had to have before embarking on a plane. I remember that Miss Large gave me a farewell party and took photos of the classroom and a photo of my two best friends, which I still have.

I have a fond memory of the ship. I had my seventh birthday party on board. The crew gave me a tin of Quality Street chocolates. How I loved those chocolates. And the last day on the ship, everyone had a big party; it was wild and lots of fun. I will never forget it. Especially the trick when the conjuror sawed someone's tummy and pretend blood spurted out of it. That has always stuck in my mind. My parents had a grand time.

When we arrived in Australia on 17 December 1969, we docked in Sydney Harbour. I saw the Opera House (which was still being built) and the big Harbour Bridge. I was very fascinated and in awe of the beauty of Sydney Harbour. We stayed at the migrant hostel, I think at Dulwich Hill.

I remember spending my first Christmas there. I was mystified because there was no snow. I said to Mum on Christmas Day, 'No snow?'

Mum replied, 'No, it's summer in Australia, no snow here.'

I think I understood but still didn't understand *why* though, as I was used to snow around Christmas.

As a young child I always wanted to know the 'why' of everything. I could not get any answers at all, as I couldn't speak properly. I found this very irritating, because I was so curious about the world around us. Luckily I had books to read. I would read my father's books about nature, animals and science. I would look into them for hours. Quite often I would ask my dad questions about his books. Usually he didn't understand me and just pointed to the pictures. We did our best to communicate, but it was hard as he has a very soft voice. I had to remind him numerous times to raise his voice (pretty daunting!). He often showed me around the garden, naming the plants and insects. He often took me and my sisters bushwalking on weekends. I loved that so much, and I loved the bush. Such a beautiful and wild land. Also, he used to take us on his small boat and we would go along the river to do some fishing and swimming. Life with him was adventurous and interesting. He still does interesting things, but he's old now and rarely goes out in his boat. His latest interest is feeding the kookaburras off our porch window. Amusing! They eat off his hands and fly away to feed their babies.

Eventually, I was integrated into a few hours in a normal-hearing class in the morning then afternoon into deaf class. I remember how scared I was with hearing children, but I managed OK with them as they were helpful. I had actually been catching up with my education; I knew I was behind them because I spent a lot of time training to speak well in the deaf unit. Then when I was twelve, I moved into full term hearing school starting sixth grade, in my sisters' school at Bankstown.

I made new friends there. A lovely girl, Christine, took me on in her group; I think she was captain of the school. I had worked hard in catching up my education; among my peers I was especially behind in English. My teacher, Mr Hill, was a very good support to me with my English.

I remember that my new friends at school couldn't believe how innocent I was. For example, I didn't know any swear words. I would get teased for that, but Christine told them to leave me alone; she was my protection and a good friend.

When the new hearing aids came in, I was ecstatic as I loathed the pocket hearing aids so much. The new ones went behind the ear. It was so cool that I could hide my hearing aids with my long hair. I was never really comfortable wearing pocket hearing aids because people would stare at them. Even worse, hearing children would tease me about them. So the new aids were a blessing.

Then I went into high school. I had special support from the

Deaf Society. A lady, I forget her name, helped with my education throughout high school. A lot of the teachers there were so supportive. Of course, I was still shy with them and sometimes I lacked confidence to ask questions but I made it through to get my School Certificate.

During Year 10 I had a private turmoil inside me. That is the reason why I left Year 11 after two months. Being a teenager isn't easy for anyone. I was no exception. I had this terrible teacher crush and I couldn't handle it, so I took a bottle of sea sickness tablets. I decided to leave school to avoid my crush and pursue a business course. Of course, I didn't tell my mother any of this, and left it that I wasn't coping with studies. By this time I had learnt to keep my feelings to myself.

There had been another private turmoil I went through, when I was in Year 9. Christine, who took me into her group, decided she couldn't be my friend any more because (the truth hurts my psyche very badly) she was so close to me that she was speaking in my deaf language, not pronouncing her words properly. Her mother had put a stop to our friendship as she wanted the best for her daughter's future. This hurt me so much that I went into a private depression. I did find another group of friends who were good to me.

This is one of the problems and disadvantages of being deaf. Throughout my entire life, I have had some close hearing friends who would imitate my speech. I realise this is normal for them as they want me to understand them, especially in one-to-one conversations. My earlier experience with my friend Christine at high school and being depressed when she rejected me, I now realise was a normal reaction to losing my best friend and there was no need to feel hurt. But I am a sensitive soul.

I prefer having close one-to-one conversations because I don't feel left out. It is a lot harder for me to follow group conversations.

But there are a lot of people I have come across who wouldn't know that I was born deaf as I speak so well, and they are amazed. I always let people know that I can't hear very well and ask them to speak clearly and slowly for me. Most of them are happy to oblige but are astounded at how well I can speak. I'm pretty proud of that. Often people ask me how I did it, as they have met other deaf people who can't speak as well as I can. I always explain that it was my mother who did a marvellous job teaching me to speak. They admire my mother for that, as well the special training at the OD Unit.

When I left high school, I went to business college. I did well there. I was stunned when I received the same high score as another girl who did Year 12. My teacher was amazed and so was the rest of the class.

After I finished my business course, I got a job at Telecom. I was elated. To my joy, I discovered there was a group of deaf ladies working there, and one deaf man too. Alas, they were all doing sign language. I knew nothing about sign language at all but I was eager to learn it. It took me a year to get it right. They invited me to join their deaf group at the Deaf Society every Friday night for social gatherings. I enjoyed being with them. I felt a sense of belonging that I hadn't felt in a long time. I spent most of my time working and socialising with them. And I saved money to travel overseas.

One of the discoveries I made about deaf people is that they have a wonderfully natural ability to read body language. I remember in high school the teacher taught about body language, though just the basic aspects. Deaf people have vastly diverse expertise with it. I was amazed. It is incredible to watch them doing it when signing.

When I was nineteen, I went to England for three months' holiday. It was lovely to see my relatives again. My cousins were all grown-up. I also saw my grandmothers, and I went to Norway to see my uncle who lives there. I went on a coach tour for two weeks; we travelled all over England, Wales and Scotland. I remember the tour guide gave me her seat because there was a mix-up with a booking. I had the best view in the front seat, the whole trip. The tour guide would stand on the stairway to make a speech. She said something really nice to me: 'I wish you were my daughter. My daughters aren't as nice as you!' I was flabbergasted with that compliment. I was just being nice to her because she had given up her seat for me; it was the least I could do.

My Aunty Pat was still living in the same house as when I left Britain when I was seven. She told me that my rabbit, Oscar, had died two years before, and I was saddened to miss him by two years. She had looked after him for me all those years, and he had lived to the ripe age of seventeen years. Wow! What was also amazing was that her next-door neighbour, Hilda, was still living there. I met her and she told me the story of when I was little; she was the one told my mother that I might be deaf.

What was even more amazing was that my Aunty Pat took me to my old school because I had wanted to search out my old school friends, Helen and Catherine. To my surprise, Miss Large was still teaching. I was shocked to see of how small she was. She was shorter than me, whereas I had memories of her being a tall lady. She was equally shocked to see how I tall I'd grown. She gave me the address of my friend, Helen. We meet up and had a lovely time together, catching up on all those lost years. I didn't see Catherine because Helen said she had become a loner. She didn't like mixing with deaf friends and was a strange girl. I was disappointed at not seeing her.

A year later, I went to America for two weeks' holiday. I went with three other women from my work. We went on a coach tour and travelled down the west coast. America was an amazing place, and I could feel the power of the country, which made my soul feel very overwhelmed by this powerful sense of energy in the atmosphere and the people. Not like Australia, or England. My experience in Mexico on the border (we went there for couple of hours) was not good. I can never forget Mexico because it was so poor. I saw kids begging to sell fruity chewing gum and mothers in rags with kids begging for money from the tourists. It was too much for my soul and I nearly fainted. My friend gave one mother some money because she was so sorry for her; it was terrible. We were all glad to get out of there and back to America. Apart from that, I enjoyed my trip. My favourite place was the Grand Canyon; it has snow there even though it is a desert place. That was amazing to me. And the scenery was so breathtaking. Beautiful.

Then I met Danny at the social group at the Deaf Society. I fell in love with his simple and uncomplicated nature and with his funny sense of humour. Danny couldn't speak at all, not one word. His world was his cars and motorbike. He loved to do up and ride his motorbike. At first I didn't understand him as he relied heavily on sign language without using any speech. Most of my partial-hearing friends used both languages: speech and sign. He was different from the rest of us. I knew my mother would abhor it; the relationship with him was not entirely what she had wanted for me. She accepted it eventually when I fell pregnant with my first son, then married Danny.

A few weeks after my son Matthew was born, he had hearing tests, and they found him to be deaf. I didn't know Danny's background (he was fostered as a baby but we discovered later his birth mother was also deaf) and I was dismayed to find my son had inherited his father's type of deafness.

The hearing clinic had talked with me about my son getting cochlear implants. That was a very, very big decision to make. The implants then were in the early stages of development and I felt it was a huge risk to take at that time. There were huge debates about the implants within the deaf community. It was twenty-five years ago when they first came out. Danny was totally dead against it, as were most of the deaf community. In the end, after much thought and discussion with my family and friends, and the experts, I made the decision that it was best for my son to have the right to choose to have cochlear implants if he wishes when he is older. My son has thanked me for the decision not to have them as a baby; he is very happy to be deaf.

Matthew went to Auslan School at North Rocks. Auslan is a sign language commonly used by deaf people as the preferred method of communication. (Before the 1960s, the School for the Deaf used finger-spelling sign language. There is a big difference.) Matthew did all right there but he wasn't happy because learning was difficult for him. Like his father, who can't read or write, I think he has inherited the same learning disorder. Or maybe he is just not interested in learning.

My communication with my son was easy compared to my mother's with me. Signing made it easy for us to understand each other. There were no major issues with that.

I have nothing against cochlear implants. I think they are a marvellous invention, but I have heard stories from people who have had them. Some say they have helped them; others say they make no difference to their hearing. One was brain-damaged by them and is now in a mental institution for life. There's always a risk factor having an operation of any sort. But I would not have them personally, simply because I just don't like the idea of cochlear implants on my head,. They look like a robot thing sticking out of your head. I prefer the hearing aids that I can take off any time I please, especially when I am tired and my head is spinning from listening through the hearing aids all day. I can really enjoy the peace and silence at the end of the day.

My favourite sounds, when I wear the hearing aids, are the birds singing. I just love hearing them and I am truly blessed that I can still hear sounds. But if ever my hearing gets worse so that I can't hear with hearing aids, I would consider cochlear implants then.

Danny and Matthew don't wear hearing aids at all. Both are very profoundly deaf and a hearing aid doesn't help them at all. Most profoundly deaf people say wearing hearing aids is like hearing very distorted noises. Hearing speech is like mumbled jargon which has no intelligence comprehension in it. It is sad, though. I was lucky that I had intensive training with listening skills and very fortunate that I had that capability to learn easily as a child.

You are probably wondering now whether these are my words, as I typed them, and you must wonder how I got to write this all down so well. When I was in high school, my English was very behind, but it was my love of reading that helped. Yes, I read a lot. A bit of a bookworm I was. I would read anything: newspapers, books of fiction, true stories and biographies, even psychology books and science. My dictionary became my best friend. My writing skills were poor, in comparison to my hearing peers, but I have worked hard to improve them over the years. I had my mother's support with my English as well. I had some private English tutoring from my teachers. (Mum has helped a bit with my grammar in this story, to make the sentences clearer in some places.)

One of my passions is my art. I went to the School of Sydney College of Painting when I was eighteen for a year's training. I just love this creative hobby; it provides very soothing therapy for my sensitive soul. I also love to play Mozart's music as I paint. When I paint, it's like I'm in another world, a world away from humdrum daily life. The stresses of life just ease away when I paint.

It was an auspicious moment in my life when I had my first solo art exhibition in 2004. It had a successful outcome and I even went on the local television news and on radio to promote my paintings. I made a speech at the exhibition opening to a number of people, including the mayor. This was the highlight of my life. I was proud of the fact I did this without the aid of a deaf interpreter to speak on my behalf. What stands out is that they reckon I have a unique style the way I do my paintings, and they were very impressed.

I was never good at sports because of my small hands and feet. I was never physically fit, always tired. I would feel bone tired in my legs and my whole body just ached all the time. That is one of the side effects of rubella, I believe. Nothing can be done for it, except to rest as much as I can. I developed arthritis as a child, mainly in my hands. Now I'm in my fifties, the arthritis is moving to my spine; one of my discs has slipped a little into the spinal cord, causing some pain in my feet and legs and a backache. I'm on painkillers, but I only take them when I need to. My doctor said it is not too bad, no need for surgery or anything like that yet. I just have to take care not to do any heavy lifting at all.

When I look back over the years at my relationships with hearing and deaf friends, I have this conflicting idea of who I am because I feel torn between my sense of belonging with deaf peers on the one hand and hearing peers on the other. With deaf peers, I can only have very simple conversations because they have very limited basic English language, whereas hearing people have a vast and diverse knowledge of the English language. I can relate to it with them, but not with my deaf peers. So I am in both worlds; it's like I am living in the middle of these two cultures. It can be a lonely experience because the deaf don't understand the hearing culture and the hearings don't understand the deaf culture. It's quite maddening: why do I understand both and they don't? It doesn't make sense. I suppose in the same way we don't always understand another country's culture. I suppose other partial-hearing people would feel the same as well, but I haven't yet tried to discuss the matter with them.

The downside of my further hearing loss is that I cannot use the phone any more. I used to be able to when my hearing was severe, but now it has become unintelligible mumbled jargon. Of course I've asked callers to slow down and speak up, but it sounds like mumbled speech. That is a loss; I miss it a lot, but not enough to get cochlear implants! I still feel scared to take the risk. Maybe in ten years' time I will get them when my hearing has virtually got no sounds, and when speech sounds like unintelligible mumbled jargon with hearing aids on. Especially if I don't hear the birds sing any more, I definitely would do it.

When I was living in Port Augusta, a small town in South Australia where I lived for about twelve years, I was the only deaf person there till I met my third husband, Winston. Winston is profoundly deaf and can't speak at all. He was trained to do one-hand finger-spelling (American-style) in the 1950s at a Sydney school.

Winston brought his five deaf friends from Adelaide to live in Port Augusta. I had to be a deaf advocate and interpreter for them. For example, doctors' appointments and church hearing friends. Once I interpreted in a court hearing as they couldn't get a professional interpreter at a moment's notice – they were based in Adelaide. Boy, that was fun! The judge was very impressed with me. I even taught the church hearing friends to learn sign language so they could communicate with the deaf. We had small classes in my home; it was a lovely experience. Mostly these church hearing friends were elderly and we would have nice morning tea and have a chat, while I was teaching.

Winston and I have one daughter, Isabel, who is hearing.

I will close off now. I do have another story to tell. It's the story of my life which has not been mentioned in this book. It's about a human tragedy which would make you all squirm and turn your toes up at. I am writing it soon.

*

After reading my mum's story about me and then my own, it became clear that we have two different experiences of dealing with deafness. Mum's experience with me is totally different from what I experienced with my own deafness. Mum's is more heartbreaking because she had no prior knowledge about deafness, whereas I lived with it.

Mum and I had a long battles and disputes in relation to the hearing and deaf worlds. It was hard for us and quite often we ended up not seeing each other for months, even years. I always felt that she didn't accept my deafness and always tried to make me like a hearing person, and she treats me like a hearing person. I did try my hardest to please her and be like a hearing person, but it was hard work. I always find it a relief to be in the company of deaf friends, though I feel I don't belong with deaf people for some reason I don't quite understand. I feel 'superior' to deaf people and I don't feel like that with hearing people; I feel normal with them.

One thing about deaf people is that they tend to repeat their story over and over and over again. I find it boring but it is not so to them. It is as if it is new news to them…amazing! But you do get used to them doing it as it is part of the deaf culture, and it is the way they are. Another thing about deaf people is that they can be really funny when they are telling you something. Sometimes I will laugh but have to hide my laughter because they can get offended! I also make mistakes when

I try to explain something. My best friend, Roberta (she is hearing), has fits of laughter when I say something on text (SMS) that I am serious about. I have to stop and think about what has made her laugh, then I look at it and I go oops!

Deaf people's mannerisms are so catching. I mean, you can end up acting like them! I suppose that's why my mother didn't want me to be like them; to her, it looks 'abnormal'. But I say to her, 'What is normal? Nowadays, everyone on earth is one crazy human being.'

And after all, hearing people say, 'It's a crazy world.'

Postscript

I received two text messages after Rachel sent me her story.

From Rachel to me:

> That story we did together made me realise how valuable you are. All the work getting me to talk properly and to listen has been really important to help me to listen and communicate with Dad. It has been worth it. He is a great dad, oh boy.

And:

> You are a wonderful mother. Don't you forget that.

When I asked Rachel to contribute her experience of what it felt like being born deaf, I was truly amazed to learn how well she could write about her childhood. She has had a turbulent and sometimes heartbreaking journey through her adult life. It is a testament to her courage and strength of character that she has managed to put those issues aside in order to share so generously and clearly her views on being deaf. She is a truly inspiring human being.

Rachel has now been a single mother for five years and lives with her father and eight-year-old daughter. She is presently doing an IT course at TAFE. She enjoys painting and is presently planning to write the second part of her life story.

At the time of publication, Rachel has made the decision to have a cochlear implant.

Margaret

Appendix

Congenital rubella syndrome (CRS) can occur in a developing foetus of a pregnant woman who has contracted rubella during her first trimester. If infection occurs 0–28 days before conception, there is a 43% chance the infant will be affected. If the infection occurs 0–12 weeks after conception, there is a 51% chance the infant will be affected.

If the infection occurs 13–26 weeks after conception there is a 23% chance the infant will be affected by the disease. Infants are not generally affected if rubella is contracted during the third trimester, or 26–40 weeks after conception. Problems rarely occur when rubella is contracted by the mother after 20 weeks of gestation and continues to disseminate the virus after birth.

It was discovered in 1941 by Australian Norman McAllister Gregg. (From Wikipedia, February 2013)

The classic triad for congenital rubella syndrome is: sensorineural deafness (58% of patients); eye abnormalities – especially retinopathy, cataract and microphthalmia (43% of patients); congenital heart disease – especially patent ductus arteriosus (50% of patients).

Other manifestations of CRS may include: spleen, liver or bone marrow problems (some of which may disappear shortly after birth); mental retardation; small head size (microcephaly); eye defects; low birth weight; thrombocytopenic purpura (presents as a characteristic blueberry muffin rash); hepatomegaly; micrognathia.

Children who have been exposed to rubella in the womb should also be watched closely as they age for any indication of the following: developmental delay; autism spectrum disorders; schizophrenia; growth retardation; learning disabilities; diabetes; glaucoma.

www.ingramcontent.com/pod-product-compliance
Ingram Content Group UK Ltd.
Pitfield, Milton Keynes, MK11 3LW, UK
UKHW041948230426
12048UKWH00008B/209